THE COURAGE TO LIVE

Donna Gustavel's Triumph Over Cerebral Palsy and Deafness

by Dan Brannan

Printed in the United States of America

First Edition - January 1997

Published by Dan Brannan Publications
P.O. Box 1708
Seneca, SC   29679

Printed by Faith Printing
Taylors, SC
Cover design by Bryan Lee and Dana Alder; cover photos by Lee Davenport; back cover by Mark Hall

Contents

About Dan Brannan

Dan Brannan has always found the inside story behind everyday people. His new book, *The Courage To Live*, is an example of that kind of story.

Throughout his career, Brannan has specialized in finding stories of people who make a difference in their communities, spotlighting what people are doing to make their communities better places to live. This approach has helped him win wide respect in the communities where he has lived.

But stories about other people are not the only ones he has written. Brannan, who has insulin-dependent diabetes, chronicled his struggle with the disease and the struggles of others in his book, *Life to the Fullest: Stories of People Coping with Diabetes*. The book is on the approved list of the American Diabetes Association and has been distributed nationally in bookstores and through the ADA's World Wide Web site.

Dan Brannan

Brannan's book *Everyday Angels* is an inspirational book focusing on average people doing extraordinary deeds. *Everyday Angels* is being distributed in several states and has attracted a national response. The book has been approved for distribution by Barnes and Noble stores and BookSmith stores throughout the Southeast. The first printing of the book was a sellout.

Dan, a native of Carrollton, Ill., located near St. Louis, graduated from Carrollton High School in 1978 and attended Eastern Illinois University in Charleston, Ill., graduating in 1982 with a degree in journalism and psychology. He began his professional career immediately at the *Shelbyville* (Ill.) *Daily Union*, where he served as sports editor and won several awards for his coverage of high school sports in central Illinois.

Three years later, Brannan joined the staff of the Thomson Newspapers *Mt. Vernon* (Ill.) *Register-News*, covering sports and was quickly promoted to sports editor. In 1988, Brannan was named managing editor of *The Standard•Democrat* in Sikeston, Mo., another Thomson paper located in the southeastern Missouri Bootheel region.

During his tenure as managing editor, he led the paper to a 20-percent increase in subscriptions, the top single percentage increase in the United States, according to the newspaper trade publication *Delivering the News,* in August 1990.

In April 1990, Thomson promoted Brannan to the managing editor position with *The Evening Telegram* in Rocky Mount, N.C., a mid-sized town located near the Raleigh-Durham-Chapel Hill Triangle area. He guided the paper to historic circulation highs and was recognized for his efforts in *Presstime* magazine and *The Financial Post*, a Toronto-based Canadian business newspaper, in 1992.

While at *The Evening Telegram*, Brannan and his staff were honored with a Thomson Newspapers Award of Excellence in 1991; a North Carolina Press Association first-place award for best investigative reporting; The Associated Press-North Carolina Parker Award for Meritorious Service; the North Carolina American Lung Association award for meritorious service in 1991-92 and again in 1992-93; and the Southern Newspaper Association Literacy Award in 1992 for the development of a weekly educational section.

Brannan left *The Evening Telegram* in the fall of 1993 to begin his own weekly newspaper, called *The Bridge*. He sold his interests in the paper in December 1994 and moved to Clemson/Seneca, S.C., to become editor of the *Journal/Tribune* and

Dan Brannan

The Messenger, leading the papers to the 1995
South Carolina Press Association's General Ex-
cellence Award in the Two- or Three-Times-
Weekly division.

Brannan led the newspaper to first place in
Community Service in 1996 and again placed
in General Excellence.

During 1995 and 1996, he guided the paper
to top honors in Best Special Section; Community Service; Best Lifestyle Section; and Business Reporting with a weekly column, *Out and
About in the Golden Corner.* The South Carolina Department of Health and Environmental
Control also honored Brannan with a 1995 state-
wide award for health promotion.

Brannan and his wife, Victoria, reside in
Upstate South Carolina.

4

Dedication

We dedicate this book to people everywhere who battle disabilities and obstacles. We especially dedicate this book to parents and children with cerebral palsy and deafness. We pray that it gives them a breath of hope that life can be relatively normal and productive, despite these problems.

We also dedicate this book to the parents of physically challenged children. It takes a very special parent to make sure that a physically challenged child grows up to have as normal a life as possible.

There have been many people who have played a role in Donna Gustavel's upbringing over the years; some of them are mentioned throughout this book. To everyone who ever had a hand in helping Donna grow and develop as a person, we wish to extend a special thank you.

5

We all know that raising such a special person is a challenge in itself. It takes extraordinary parenting skills to raise a physically challenged person. Without the patience and love that these parents show, these children would not be able to rise above their handicaps and show the world their true beauty.

It is to all these individuals that this book is expressly dedicated.

Introduction

One day at the Kourthouse Fitness Center in Keowee Key, S.C., I looked up and saw an amazing physical sight.

I saw a lady, who apparently had some major physical limitations, giving it her all on the StairMaster leg machine.

The lady's name was Donna Gustavel. I don't remember when or how we first communicated, but I was captivated by her courage, determination and character.

I watched Donna at the Kourthouse many times before I actually introduced myself. When I first met her in the fall of 1994, life was not a bowl of cherries for me. I had developed diabetes and was going through several other difficulties in my life. I can remember how inspiring Donna was when I was doing my workouts.

I don't know how many times I've seen her fall off the StairMaster. Her cerebral palsy affects her coordination and her ability to stand stationary. Each time I saw her get up from a fall, I think it gave me the inspiration that maybe having diabetes and being insulin-dependent wasn't such a bad fate, after all.

I had been fortunate to have 33 years without any major physical difficulties, whereas Donna had spent her entire life battling deafness, cerebral palsy and many muscular and skeletal problems.

Before mid-March, 1995, I hadn't spoken much to Donna's father, Don, and I hadn't met Donna's mother, Marcelle. Don and Donna worked out side-by-side each time they came to the Kourthouse. Hand-in-hand, I saw them come in and do their workout. Many times, I would also see them walking out hand-in-hand.

I told Donna's story in the *Journal/Tribune* newspaper of Seneca, S.C., in the March 22, 1995, issue.

My column headline that day read "Donna Gustavel shows courage every step of the way." The column started like this:

"Each step in Keowee Key resident Donna Gustavel's 41-year-old life has required more courage than most could possibly imagine.

"Because of cerebral palsy, Donna wasn't able to even take her first steps until she was 5. Cerebral palsy is a disease which affects the central nervous system, especially during birth, and is usually characterized by spastic paralysis.

"Donna could have lived a normal life, especially if her condition had been diagnosed properly at birth.

"Donna had an Rh blood factor and should have immediately had her blood exchanged, but by the time it was done, it was too late. She already had damage.

"She developed not only cerebral palsy, but was also born deaf. Life expectancy for someone in Donna's condition is only about 20 years; she has doubled that."

After the column appeared, Donna received cards and letters from all over the country, including a note from my golfing favorite, Jack Nicklaus. "The Golden Bear" responded on April 17, 1995, with a letter that said:

"Dear Donna,
"Thanks for your nice note and the copy of Dan Brannan's great article. I enjoyed it a lot and agree with him wholeheartedly!

"It has been awhile since our paths have

crossed, but I am happy to know you're doing well - and still making those chocolate chip cookies!

"Say hello to your parents for me, and keep up the good work at the gym.

**"Your friend,
Jack Nicklaus."**

Donna also appeared in chapter 5 of my book, *Everyday Angels*, under the title, "The Courage To Live." The chapter began with a quote from Marcelle, which read: "Donna has taught me a lot by being kind, gentle, loving and understanding. She is just a marvelous person, very thoughtful."

After *Everyday Angels*, I took my time pondering what my next book project would be. I had always wanted to do a biography and decided that I had to tell Donna's complete story.

I believe that Donna is an inspiration for the 1990s, much like Helen Keller was during the early part of the 20th century. Keller was born in 1880 in Tuscumbia, Ala., but when she was 19 months old, she suffered from an acute illness that nearly killed her and left her deaf and blind. Thanks to an incredible teacher, Annie Sullivan, Keller graduated from Radcliffe College in 1904 and dedicated her life to helping the blind and handicapped.

Keller died in 1968. Her burial urn is located in the National Cathedral in Washington. Keller's early years were chronicled in the classic Broadway play and Oscar-winning film, *The Miracle Worker.*

Donna, like Helen Keller, has devoted her life to helping other physically challenged children.

What follows is the story of one of the most courageous persons I have ever met in my life. What she has endured and triumphed over will inspire you. I know it certainly inspired me.

Prologue

God's Child

It isn't what you say or do.
What's on the outside doesn't count.
It's in the heart - if it is true.
Love, happiness, contentment will mount.

I saw this happen before my own eyes.
It started when she was little in size.
Her heart had grown bigger than her height.
She loves you and you with all her might.

She cannot hear, nor can she talk
She even has a funny walk.
But there's a twinkle in her eye.
She makes you feel you're 10 feet high.

Feeling depressed and a little down?
She'll make you smile instead of frown.
She's sharp, quick and smart as can be.
With a sense of humor and personality.

The Courage To Live

Do I love her? Indeed, I do
When you meet her, you will too.

Marcelle Gustavel,
writing about her daughter Donna

Chapter 1

A Profile in Courage

Frequently, Donna Gustavel and her father, Don, load up the car with their gym bags and drive about a mile down the road to the Kourthouse Fitness Center, located in Keowee Key, S.C.

The Gustavels go through a workout routine that would probably tire Arnold Schwarzenegger.

The Gustavels believe one of the key factors in keeping Donna healthy has been being active and staying physically fit through all her 41 years of life. Born with cerebral palsy and deafness, Donna today stands 4-foot-11 and weighs 70 pounds. For enduring all of her physical problems, surgeries and obstacles along the way, Donna is an amazing physical specimen.

Ed Rumsey, in his 60s, is a pretty imposing physical specimen himself. A former Air Force officer, Rumsey manages the Kourthouse. When he initially opened the club, the Gustavels were among his first customers.

"She always had a smile on her face," Rumsey recalled. "I got to know her better by visiting with her while she exercised. She has tremendous determination. She starts her workout by climbing on the StairMaster at a low level. To watch her sway her crooked bones up and down for about 30 minutes is about as inspiring as it gets."

At the gym, Donna moves from the StairMaster to the leg machine and does leg extensions, working her quadricep muscles and knees for about 15-20 minutes. From there, she goes to the situp board and does curls. "One day, I watched and I counted 73 curls, which is amazing for someone with her physical challenges," Rumsey said. "I think anyone would be very amazed to watch her work out.

"I think a lot of people in her position would accept her type of condition as fate and not attempt to do anything about it. Donna is a very intelligent person. She collects aluminum cans from people around the Keowee area and pays for everything she does. She doesn't want anyone to feel sorry for her."

Often, Donna falls off the StairMaster. In fact, I have been present several times when she has fallen because of loss of muscular coordination. Every time Donna falls off, though, she gets right back up and gets back on the machine.

"She never wants to quit," Rumsey said. "She works out the entire time her father is at the Kourthouse. She is in perpetual motion. If Don can't come, her mother brings her and waits patiently. She never stops and keeps on going and going."

Marcelle knows when she takes Donna to the gym, it will be a long wait. Donna's workout routine takes about two-and-a-half hours to finish. "Don is in remarkable shape for someone who is age 71, just 11 days older than me," Marcelle said. "Donna works just as hard as Don does. Don and Donna are buddies. They enjoy their workout time together."

Donna appreciates the time Rumsey has taken with her, especially after one incident that took place when Donna was in her early 20s and living in Atlanta. Marcelle attempted to take Donna to join one of the major chain health clubs there. Management said that it would be no problem having her join, and Donna paid her initial fees. Marcelle even purchased exercise outfits for her.

When Donna showed up to exercise, management changed their minds and refused to let Donna work out, fearing injury. Marcelle said she would have signed any release in order for Donna to work out, but the chain would not allow Donna to use their facilities.

"Before I knew it, our check was returned to us in the mail," Marcelle said. "It broke my heart and Donna's. I was very upset with them and the way it was handled. They didn't give Donna a chance."

Rumsey, like many of his Keowee Key friends, has fallen in love with Donna's chocolate chip cookies. He describes them as very moist and tasty. "She loads them with a lot of chocolate and takes a lot of time to make sure the cookies are outstanding," Rumsey said.

Rumsey is a firm believer that Donna's exercise program has extended her life and made her life more enjoyable. Many cerebral palsy patients end up in a wheelchair by age 6 or 7 and have a life expectancy of about 20 years. Donna has lived well beyond - in fact, about double the time - that most cerebral palsy patients live.

Rumsey has learned sign language so he can communicate with her.

"If Donna could speak, you would find a very intelligent person and a person who is aware of what is going on," Rumsey said. "Many people who have this type of disease or other crippling diseases become vegetables and believe that is their fate, but not Donna. She is a very nice young lady."

Rumsey understands most of Donna's sign language, especially after reading some material on it. He says that if he gets lost during the communication process, he has her write down what she is trying to say.

A few years back, Rumsey put on a racquetball tournament at the facility. Donna volunteered to help, getting drinks for everyone and helping at the front counter. Rumsey said he was impressed with how Donna handled herself that day and how she took charge of various tasks.

"If people who have a bad knee or a few other aches and pains could see her in action, they would never have a gripe," Rumsey said. "Her willpower is just amazing. I used to be a fighter pilot, and I have said this before, but I will say it again: I would let her fly on my wing anytime."

Chapter 2

Life Begins

Feb. 16, 1954, to most people, was an average, routine day. But to Don and Marcelle Gustavel, this was no ordinary day.

Their second daughter, Donna, was born on this day - one month and a day premature - at Children's Hospital in San Francisco. Don had started in industrial sales two years earlier for The Bowser Company, an Indiana-based firm.

Don vividly remembers the day Donna was born - with an Rh factor. "They had a lack of knowledge of Rh factors back then," Don recalled. An Rh factor is any one of inheritable antigen factors in the red blood cells, a lack of which can cause a severe - sometimes fatal - reaction in infants. "Today, a blood exchange would be automatic at birth.

"She was jaundiced before they realized there

was a problem. One doctor even commented she would be a fair blonde because of the jaundice. They realized too late that a blood exchange was needed. The blood was exchanged on the third day, but the damage had already been done.

"The damage was at the receiving end of the brain. Fortunately, the damage did not affect her intellect."

Marcelle remembered that she was frightened at first because Donna wasn't crying at birth like her first child, Michele, did. "The doctor reassured me she was fine; he hit her little bottom, and I heard a whimper," Marcelle said. "Shortly after that, he showed her to me. She was, indeed, beautiful, delicate and possessed a tranquility that told me she was God's child.

"In a matter of three days, her dark hair became very light, and her translucent skin became yellow. Just as quickly, she turned from a beautiful baby to a very old-appearing person, one that was wrinkled. I could hardly believe my eyes. They told me she cried all the time. The doctor was very busy running all types of tests, and the final decision was made - a complete exchange of blood.

"We were told that if she survived the procedure, she would be fine. How very naive we were. The damage had already been done."

When one thinks about it, only 72 hours separated Donna from living a normal life. If only the doctors had seen the need for the exchange earlier, things might have been different. Still, despite the setbacks, the Gustavels had much to be pleased about.

"My husband and I were very happy. We were a family of four, with two little girls very close in age."

Marcelle believed Don was a big help during Donna's recovery in the hospital, constantly going back and forth from his job to see her.

"Father had a lot of blood tests to see what went wrong," Donna said. "He helped in the diagnosis of my palsy. I realize today that a lack of blood circulating did the damage to me at birth."

Marcelle remembered when the first shock came after coming home. Donna had trouble keeping milk down and had vomited slightly. "I told the doctor of a peculiar reaction she had," Marcelle recalled. "It was then that the doctor told me that he had been waiting for such a sign, and that our baby had cerebral palsy.

"The heartbreak we both suffered back then could never be expressed in words."

However, that wasn't the end of the Gustavels' troubles. They were in for another shock. "I discovered that she never responded to sound,"

Marcelle said. "Then tests proved she was deaf. The first six months of her life, I had to feed her every two hours around the clock. The second six months, she cried all night, every night."

Almost overnight, her personality started to develop, and there were signs of a sense of humor. "She was just a little over a year old when she attended a nursery school for spastic children. I was shown how to exercise her legs daily, how to motivate the use of her arms and hands. She played in coffee grounds and flour, she felt the sand and the ocean, the wet grass and dry grass.

"I showed her everything inside the house. Outside, she touched everything and anything."

Marcelle remembered that her friends and family were fearful of holding Donna because she wiggled so much.

At this point, the Gustavels knew they had plenty to handle. What they didn't know was what kind of fighter they had for a daughter.

Chapter 3

What Makes
Her "Special"?

Donna Gustavel has often been described as a "special" person. Just how special she is comes to light once one realizes the kinds of obstacles she has overcome in her life.

Donna was born with cerebral palsy, which is a phrase used to cover a wide variety of problems that affect a person's ability to move and maintain posture and balance. Generally, CP is caused by a brain injury that takes place during the birth process, whether it is before a child is born, during the actual birth or following birth.

The cause of the brain damage can be a failure of the brain to develop fully during gestation or because of neurological damage to the brain during development. Quite often, brain injuries can be caused by a lack of oxygen to the brain during gestation or during the birth process or because of bleeding inside the brain.

In most cases, the area of the brain affected is the one that controls muscle movement. However, other problems can occur, such as mental retardation, seizures, language problems, learning disabilities and hearing problems. According to the latest statistics, about two children out of every 1,000 born in the United States have CP to some degree. In fact, more people in this nation have CP than any other developmental disability, including Down's syndrome, epilepsy and autism.

While those with mild cases of CP can recover by the time they reach school age, CP is usually a lifelong disability. The severity of the condition can affect a child's learning process and his or her ability to perform necessary tasks to care for him or herself.

One way of telling if a child has CP has to do with the state of the child's muscle tone, which is the amount of tension or resistance to movement in a muscle. Since the damaged area of the brain in CP often controls muscle tone, the child can be affected in different ways.

In those with high muscle tone (also called spasticity), movements are often stiff and awkward; symptoms include an exaggerated arch of the back and stiff extension of the legs.

Those with low muscle tone have trouble maintaining positions without support because muscles cannot contract enough; they have trouble sitting or standing up straight because the muscles cannot support them against gravity.

Children with a combination of low and high tone (called fluctuating tone) often have low tone at rest, but high tone when active. Sitting up straight, for example, may be no problem, but reaching for an object may become impossible because the muscle groups in the shoulders and arms, for example, may tighten up.

There are three types of CP: pyramidal, or spastic, CP; extrapyramidal, or choreoathetoid, CP; and mixed-type CP. Symptoms of pyramidal CP include exaggerated stretch reflexes, in which limbs extend with a jerk much stronger than normal; ankle clonus, in which calf and foot muscles contract in a rapid and rhythmical pattern; positive babinski, when a child's toes extend and fan out rather than flex when a foot is stroked; a tendency for a child to develop contractures, or abnormal shortening, of the muscles and tendons around a joint; and persistent primitive reflexes, in which early reflexes in response to simple stimuli persist for months or years longer than what is usual.

In extrapyramidal CP, severe damage to the area of the brain controlling simple movements can cause problems with simple tasks, such as speaking, feeding, reaching and other vital skills needed for survival. Instead, the child affected often displays involuntary movements, movements that can grow more severe as time goes on.

Emotional stress, fear or anxiety can cause the movements to become more pronounced or severe. The movements often fade away, however, while the child is asleep.

Mixed-type CP patients often exhibit combined symptoms of the first two types, often because of damage to the two areas of the brain that control muscle movements and tone. The child's spasticity is more noticeable between the ages of 9 months and 3 years.

Needless to say, CP affects different children in different ways. There is no one set pattern of treatment or training for those with CP. In general, however, most programs will include a therapeutic exercise program for the child's condition. Physical therapists, occupational therapists and speech pathologists will often team up to provide a child with the best care and training possible under the supervision of the attending physician.

According to *The New Webster Dictionary of*

the English Language, deafness is defined as a person who is "wholly or partly deprived of the sense of hearing." In Donna's case, her cerebral palsy caused her deafness from the time she was born. Donna never responded to sound, and tests proved that she was deaf.

Despite her condition, Donna has been able to communicate through the use of sign language. Donna's main problem, like others with cerebral palsy, is that, at times, her condition makes it difficult for her to be able to sign clearly because of the deterioration of the muscles needed to be able to use sign language.

To see Donna go about her life despite these severe challenges is remarkable. It is amazing what she has accomplished and what she has done in her 40-plus years of life, a lifespan far beyond what most people in her condition would have a right to expect.

Chapter 4

One Day, One Step at a Time

Raising a child is a difficult job, but when someone tells you your child will face all sorts of problems as he or she grows up, the prospects can be devastating.

Perhaps that was what the Gustavels had to look forward to when Donna was just 10 months old. A series of tests conducted on Donna at the nursery school she was attending revealed to the doctors that Donna's intellect would, more than likely, not exceed the level of a 3-year-old.

Marcelle remembered seeing red when she heard the psychologist's words that day.

"Donna showed Don and me signs of being capable of much more than that," Marcelle said. "You just had to be with her to understand. In many of the tests she has had over the years, the doctors said she likely would have been a very brilliant person. She is very, very smart. She takes

care of her own bank account and she has a remarkable memory.

"She remembers everyone's face and remembers everything that happens to her. She may not
remember someone by name, but she will remember where they met and recall the face."

One of the Gustavels' biggest scares took place
in San Francisco when Donna was 2 years old.
Donna, being curious like any 2-year-old, found
a nearby hot coffee pot and turned it over. The
hot liquid spilled on her and burned her arms and
back. The burns ended up being third-degree.

"I cut Donna's clothes off, and Don called the
doctor," Marcelle recalled. "We wound up having to give her a shot of morphine for the pain.
She didn't have to have surgery, but she had to be
given cold baths for the skin.

"We were so careful after that. Her cerebral
palsy made things very restrictive, and we had to
respect those restrictions."

One of the highlights of Donna's young
life was appearing on a Bay Area television
station to promote a San Francisco Children's
Hospital program about early birth defects,
including multiple handicaps.

"She was about a year-and-a-half old
when she appeared on the show," Marcelle
said. "We were very proud of her. She has

always been a ham for the camera. She has always been an extrovert."

Don's biggest worry was not the fact that Donna was deaf. "I feared she would never walk," Don said. "There was a lot of uncertainty about her future and about how we could best help her. There just weren't many programs available back then for those with multiple handicaps."

Marcelle, like Don, feared Donna would never walk. As a rule, children usually take their first steps around their first birthday. Donna took her first steps at age 5. Marcelle says that if it hadn't been for the help of occupational and physical therapists who worked on her case, Donna likely would have never walked.

"It was a thrill to see her take her first steps," Marcelle said. Don also said it was one of his greatest thrills to see his daughter walk for the first time.

Communication was the next hurdle to overcome for Donna and her parents. Amazingly, the Gustavels never took a sign language course to help them communicate with Donna, but learned sign language through Donna's teaching and books of their own. "We never had a true sign language course," Marcelle said. "Donna's will was very strong when she was young. She was a very easy student to teach."

Donna easily grasped the sign-language alphabet and learned phrases and other signs quickly.

Don remembers her physical handicaps kept her from flashing signs as proficiently as people who were only deaf. "She was too slow for deaf people," Don said. "They definitely went too fast for her."

Donna remembered one school principal signing so gracefully, she almost resembled a ballet dancer. "It depends on the person's method whether or not I can understand the signs," Donna said.

Marcelle and Don instituted a philosophy that they would take things one day and one step at a time. "I think I was so busy doing what I had to do, taking care of my two children, I didn't have time to feel any fear," Marcelle said.

Chapter 5

School Days, School Days

Most kids today start school at a very young age, getting the basics down even before they start kindergarten.

Donna was no exception, but the school she attended, El Portal School in San Mateo, Calif., was no ordinary school.

This school was a place where children with multiple handicaps could learn not only reading, writing and math, but also many of the life skills most of us take for granted.

Marcelle believes the El Portal experience was one of the keys to Donna having such a successful life. "If she hadn't been there, I don't think she would have materialized into the kind of person she turned out to be," Marcelle said. "I definitely think it was the key to her later success.

"We were very fortunate to be in such a progressive state like California; they are not afraid to try new ideas. They had a lot of knowledge of people with multiple handicaps."

Marcelle and Don have always transported Donna to wherever she had to go. Marcelle remembered driving through the well-known San Francisco fog on the way to and from Donna's school.

First, the Gustavels looked at the California School for the Deaf in Berkeley, but the school would not accept Donna because of her multiple handicaps. The Gustavels also tried to send her to a school in Burlingame, Calif., but again, problems cropped up.

One of those problems was a bus driver who was nervous about Donna boarding his bus with a helmet on. The other children attending Burlingame were only deaf. Donna could not keep up with the other kids in classes such as physical education and could not perform many of the tasks the other children could do.

"It was too much of a strain on her," Marcelle said. "These children were deaf, but very physically capable."

Eventually, the Gustavels pulled Donna from Burlingame, and she went to school at El Portal.

One of Donna's favorite teachers at El Portal was Mary Bond, with whom the

Gustavels still correspond. When asked about her, Donna had a big smile.

"She was a very good teacher," Donna said. "I loved her. She taught me very well. There is a strong bond between the two of us."

Donna said the teachers taught her many things at El Portal. "I was very tiny, and they held my hand and put it in things such as coffee grounds and many other things so I could experience different forms of touch," Donna recalled.

Marcelle said that the El Portal staff also worked with her on her arm movements and the development of her eyes to overcome some of her muscular difficulties.

Don always believed El Portal was a very good school for her, but still restrictive because of a lack of training for deaf students. "They had great groups of teachers," he said. "They had both occupational and physical therapy, which was helpful for Donna."

During Donna's elementary school days, she met one of her best friends in life, Laura. She was her next-door neighbor.

One of Donna's important youthful moments came when she was about 12 years old. There was a birthday party for both Donna and Laura. The two girls got matching dresses.

"The girls were very good pals," Marcelle said.

"We were very close to Laura's family; they were our next-door neighbors. When we moved to Tennessee, Laura stayed a month with us. Laura is about 36 today; she and Donna remain good friends."

Donna's kind heart started to develop while she was at El Portal. One time, Donna was around a little girl who was constantly sick with seizures. Donna often held the girl in her arms and showed her love and care.

Academically, Donna strived for A's and got them. She brought schoolwork home and would work for hours perfecting her spelling with Marcelle at her side.

Donna said that the things she remembers the most of her El Portal experience was playing basketball, being a pom-pon girl, being the school's dominos queen and singing in the choir. Marcelle recalled that Donna got right up and sang with the group when the time came.

Donna's graduation from El Portal on June 10, 1969, was a big day for the family. Now, it was time to leave the elementary years behind and move on to the higher-level academic training. Donna wore a beautiful white dress that day, and many friends attended the ceremonies.

"We were very proud, and very sad, on graduation day," Marcelle said. "We hated to leave a lot of those people behind; they had done so much for Donna.

"Leaving the people behind was the hardest part of leaving El Portal. When Donna left, perhaps the nicest gift she received was a diamond heart chain from the faculty."

Chapter 6

On the Move

Following Donna's graduation from El Portal School, her father Don was transferred to Cookville, Tenn., as general sales manager of Keene Corporation's filtration division, which had bought out his previous employer, The Bowser Company. Don had risen to regional manager for the western United States at Bowser before the Keene takeover.

Don's duties included selling industrial filtration and pollution control equipment for many heavy industries. He traveled throughout the nation.

Don took his family to Tennessee when he was transferred. Donna quickly became a volunteer at a local school for deaf children. Marcelle attempted to enroll Donna in school in Knoxville, Tenn., but found it again very difficult for Donna physically. Donna also had a scary experience with a 50-year-old mentally handicapped person.

"The woman had grabbed Donna and squeezed her for a long period of time, and she couldn't get away," Marcelle said. "She started screaming for me, and she didn't want to go back to that school after that incident." It took the Gustavels some time to get over that incident.

Still, one of Donna's fondest memories of Tennessee was having a pony named Lightning. She had a saddle and the works for the horse. She has always had a love of animals. Her sister, Michele, also had a horse who was very gentle with Donna.

"Animals are very sensitive, and horses especially are sensitive to a handicapped person's needs," Marcelle said. "Michele's horse would walk gently and turn gently with Donna. She loved riding horses."

Eleanor Sadler and Glenn and Ellen Crocker became good friends with Donna while she lived in Cookville.

"We went to church together and became good friends," Sadler said. "I have known her for about 20 years. She is a very smart person; she does have handicaps, but there is nothing wrong with her brain. Her parents have helped her so much. I don't know if I could get through what she has been through. She is a brave child."

The Crockers now live in Cincinnati, but Donna has stayed in contact with them. "We are extremely close," Ellen Crocker said. "I have always loved her, and she has loved me."

Next, the family moved to Baton Rouge, La., where Don was a partner in a boat store that serviced tugboats near the Mississippi River. Donna attended the Louisiana School for Spastic Children, which was a help for her.

"Things went very well at that school," Marcelle said. "All her teachers were intelligent and understanding. Donna did well and was well-liked there."

Don then became an Atlanta partner in the same business he had worked for Keene. The company covered seven Southeastern states. He concluded his working career as president of Liquid Handling Specialists in Atlanta.

When the Gustavels moved to Atlanta, they enrolled Donna at the Georgia School for the Deaf in Rome, Ga. Donna, as always, did well at the school and was a well-liked student. She especially liked her principal at that school.

Don felt the environment was much better at GSD than it had been at the Tennessee school.

Her biggest moment in her academic career came when she graduated from GSD on May 23, 1974. Both Don and Marcelle remembered

Donna's graduation as one of the highlights of her life.

"She was acknowledged on the stage," Marcelle said. "The principal talked highly of her that night. She was given a rose, and she broke down and cried. It was a very touching ceremony."

Donna always said she loved the school. "I learned a lot there," Donna recalled. "I got along with everyone. It was really sad when I had to leave the school. I especially was sad to leave Principal Highnote."

When Donna reached age 20, the fact that she no longer was a little girl began to sink in for the Gustavels. The years of training and hard work were the reasons. She was now a self-sufficient person, able to perform many physical tasks. Her physical handicaps had become secondary to her deafness.

Marcelle recalled being frightened of what Donna's future might be. "We had learned to live day-to-day, but as I aged, I found it a little difficult," Marcelle said. "We had so much help and guidance when she was young, but now, we wondered who we would turn to now that she was not so young."

Donna knew that following her graduation, she would never drive a car, have her own apartment, have real friends socially, have a boyfriend, get married and have children. She decided that since she could not have these things, she would become successful in her work.

Donna wanted responsibilities and wanted to be needed and depended upon. "Donna had always been a responsible person, very dependable and devoted," Marcelle said. "So much went on in that mind of hers; she had so many good ideas and thought of things I would never think of. She had such a good temperament; it was very easy for her to get along with others."

Donna's school years had come to an end. It was now time for her to get on with her life.

Chapter 7

Smooth Operator

M ost people in Donna's condition have to undergo an operation or two. Donna, in fact, has had *eight* surgeries over the course of her 40-plus years, beginning with the life-saving blood exchange operation she underwent right after she was born.

Soon after, Donna had oral surgery to correct a lack of tooth buds in her mouth; after that came the incident in which she was burned (she nearly underwent a skin graft for that). That was followed by an operation on her neck to place a bone from her hip in that area for stability.

She has had two cysts removed, plus two ovarian operations and has had plates and screws installed in the back of her neck, an operation which took some seven hours to complete.

"Donna was dropping her head prior to the

plates and screws being put in," Marcelle said about this 1992 operation. "The plates and screws helped bring her head up. This was a very touch-and-go surgery.

"It was not easy; she was in a lot of pain. I had to bathe and feed her. She couldn't get her hands to move. After we got home, Donna slept upstairs for a month while I slept downstairs. She was on a lot of pills and medication while she recovered."

In 1980, Dr. Julian Fuerst removed her ovaries, a procedure that was very difficult to perform. Marcelle stayed with Donna throughout the process, with Don providing relief when he could.

In 1984, Donna had neck surgery at DeKalb Medical Center in Atlanta under the direction of Dr. Roy Vandiver, a neurosurgeon in metro Atlanta. "Donna was very receptive to surgery and cooperative," Marcelle remarked. "She always went in to get better."

Dr. Vandiver works out of Atlanta Neurosurgical Associates, located at DeKalb Medical Center in suburban Atlanta. He has been a neurosurgeon in metro Atlanta since 1967.

Vandiver remembered doing the cervical fusion for Donna back in 1984. Donna, at the time, had spinal problems complicated by other problems created by her cerebral palsy. Through the years, Vandiver and Donna have continued their doctor-patient relationship, but they have also become good friends.

"We became friends after she was a patient of mine," Vandiver said. "She is an inspiration to be around. She keeps going on, no matter what. I see her on a regular basis and correspond with her through cards. I see her yearly."

Dr. Vandiver also helped set up Donna's 1992 neck operation by Dr. Charles L. Branch at Baptist Medical Center in Winston-Salem, N.C. Vandiver has deep admiration for Donna.

"I have never had a patient with as many physical problems and people still love to be around so much," Vandiver said. "She comes into our office, and everyone loves her. She is very friendly. She is always interested in what everyone is doing.

"Donna handles adversity well. She realizes that she has limitations to what she can accomplish physically, but she keeps climbing the next mountain."

Vandiver, like many others, is a fan of Donna's chocolate chip cookies. In fact, the staff in DeKalb literally fight over the delicacies when Donna brings them.

"I see people every day who have physical problems that aren't even close to Donna's problems from day one," Vandiver said, "but they do much, much less with their lives. Her philosophy is basically 'I know I've got a problem; let's do what we have to do and go on from there.'"

Vandiver is also impressed with Don, Marcelle and Michele, and the support they have given Donna. In fact, he believes Donna would have never made it as far as she did without her parents' tender loving care.

People have always been kind to Donna in the hospital. When she was in Winston-Salem having surgery, Dr. Vandiver sent her flowers. Atlanta-area hairdresser Ray Stephens has also always loved Donna and once came to her home after surgery, cutting her hair and bringing a dozen roses. Donna's biggest surprise after an operation came when father Don came toting what Marcelle called "the biggest Snoopy ever made" from their car to the hospital. "It was sticking about halfway out of our car, and when Don brought it into the hospital, everyone took notice," Marcelle said.

Dr. James Hanahan, a physician in Seneca, S.C., has been the Gustavel's family doctor for more than a decade. Donna has, he says, a little spunk inside of her that is not present in most people.

"I can't tell you everything she has done in her life," Hanahan said, "but I know that spark is still there today. She has so many neuromuscular deficiencies; some persons would take difficulties like Donna has and not try to do anything with them."

Dr. Hanahan recalls one time when, while at Keowee Key for a function, he saw her out with her parents on the putting green at the local golf course. Hanahan believes Donna is a remarkable physical specimen.

"She lives with pain in the neck area and in various muscles," he said. "When you see someone with that many physical problems, it makes your own problems seem insignificant. Donna keeps her muscle strength balanced.

"For cerebral palsy patients, muscle balance can be a real problem. It can especially be a problem if the other muscles aren't that strong. I think it is very inspirational to see what Donna has done with her life."

What Hanahan loves the most about Donna is her beautiful smile. "Because of the palsy, her smile is somewhat distorted, but you can see deep down, looking at her, what a beautiful smile it is," Hanahan said.

The Gustavels are very pleased with Dr. Hanahan's care of Donna and believe he has been a big help in keeping her healthy during their time in South Carolina.

Donna's exercise regimen has also played a big role in her remaining healthy, Vandiver believes. "Donna is an example for others to follow," Vandiver said. "If they could make a serum out of her enthusiasm, desire and positive attitude and could inoculate the whole world with it, we would have a better world."

Chapter 8

Finding a Niche

The Coralwood Center in DeKalb County, Ga., has never been the same since Donna left it on Nov. 8, 1985. She began volunteering at the facility, a place for children with learning disabilities in the DeKalb County school system, soon after her graduation from the Georgia School for the Deaf in 1974.

Her volunteer work at Coralwood answered the Gustavels' hopes and prayers. "When we moved to Atlanta, we wondered what we were going to do for Donna," Marcelle recalled. "I heard on the radio about a person who did sign language for a class."

Marcelle then got the idea about approaching Coralwood and asking them if they would allow Donna to volunteer. One class, taught by Gennie Howes, gave Donna the opportunity to work in a classroom.

"She worked in my classroom for a number of years," Howes recalled. "She started in 1974 and was an assistant to an aide in my classroom. She helped with the children and helped with the different jobs that needed to be done. Eventually, she worked as a library aide."

Howes described Donna as a joy to be around.

"Donna was a very positive influence on the children," Howes said. "The children loved her. She was a ray of sunshine in the classroom. She was very enthusiastic and ambitious and was willing to do anything I needed."

Donna was not one of the first to rush out of the school each day. In fact, she always stayed behind, working with the children.

Howes believes one of the reasons she was paired with Donna was that she knew a little sign language. Donna volunteered and dedicated her time at the center for a year in the hopes she could be employed.

Donna did all kinds of things during her first year, working with children with matrix cards, puzzles and countless ideas to help improve the children's learning. "Donna worked with the children, and they just loved her," Marcelle said. "She always worked eight hours a day and was so personal with the kids.

"Gennie Howes let Donna do a lot of things

to help the children."

Donna could often be found on the playground or assisting the loading of children on buses at the school. She also worked in the lunchroom area, helping to coordinate the cafeteria lunch schedules. Each day, Marcelle was tending to Donna, taking her to and from work and often staying behind to help her with her school tasks.

Howes and Principal Angela Edwards, along with a number of other people, thought so much of Donna that they recommended her for a paid state aide position after her first year. Mary Janet Hardin on the board of education also played an important part in Donna getting her break.

"I was extremely proud of her when she was able to have her own money, have an occupation and a career," Howes said. "The fact that she could earn her own livelihood, at whatever level she could without hearing, speaking and her muscular movement problems speaks for itself."

Howes views Donna as a tremendous inspiration. "She overcame so many physical limitations, along with speech and hearing difficulties," Howes said. "She still has a bright smile, her positive spirit and her will. Donna is such a sweet soul."

Don was proud of Donna for volunteering and earning her stripes. "The Coralwood job was actually a result of her mother's tenacity and dedication to get something for Donna," Don said. "Once she got the break, Donna's dedication and perseverance showed, and she won the confidence of all with whom she worked.

"She also became a sounding board for all the teachers with their personal problems."

Donna's spirit got her a job and over the next few years, her spirit would help make Coralwood one of the happiest schools in all of Georgia.

Chapter 9

A Helping Hand

In more than a decade at the Coralwood Center, Donna's infectious spirit and work habits made her an unforgettable part of the facility to faculty, staff and students alike.

Donna accomplished this in many ways, including helping re-establish a library in a part of the center that had previously been closed. The library became one of her biggest projects, and she made sure the books were returned after they were borrowed and put in to their proper place on the shelves.

Marcelle recalled that every book had a distinct place in the library. "She was pretty strict about making sure everyone got their books back," she said. Marcelle worked closely with Donna to make sure the library was a success.

"Donna made sure the books were put out a certain way so they would show up on their shelf. During the holiday season, she would also put certain books out related to the season."

When Donna retired, Coralwood put a plaque up on the door of the library commemorating her work.

Donna has always loved the holiday season and constantly demonstrated that at Coralwood. "During Christmas, she had special gifts for all the children in her classrooms," Marcelle said. "If the class was especially wonderful, they got a special gift. All the gifts came out of her salary. During Halloween, Donna would make sure they all got candy after lunch and would often be in costume to cheer their spirits up.

"Donna was never late for work. Donna would get up and always be ready to go. She only missed a few days out of all the time she spent there because she was sick."

"I got tremendous joy out of working with the children," Donna said. "When they were wrong, I disciplined them, and when they needed a hug, I hugged them. I felt I had a great relationship with the teachers and the parents.

"Some of the kids were hard to handle, and they all had different problems. I loved them all."

Gennie Howes, the teacher Donna worked with at Coralwood, remarked that "Donna gave a lot to this school, the children and the community. The children loved her. She was instinctive and intuitive with them. She is a very special person.

"She definitely gave a lot back to the school. It was nothing but an outpouring of love. She is contagious in her ability to elicit love. She loves everyone. Whenever she saw a need or someone who needed help in the classroom, she didn't hesitate to bring in her own money. That takes a very special person."

When Donna retired, Howes said she was very sad to see her go, but respected her decision, knowing she wanted to go with her parents to the Keowee Key, S.C., area.

"I just feel privileged and honored to have had her in my classroom," Howes said, "and for her to be my associate. If anyone was having a down or blue day, she would be so sensitive to you. She is a very sensitive person; she would always pick you up when you needed it."

Principal Angela Edwards also remembered Donna's efforts fondly.

"Everyone at the school loved her," she said. "It seems like she could almost read your mind. She always seemed to know what you were saying and would start laughing at things that were funny. She was a very joyful person.

"DeKalb County (Ga.) hired her as an assistant. She did a lot of different tasks, from putting out juice and milk in the cafeteria to fixing the tables with napkins and utensils. She and another person met the children at the bus and she had other tasks, as well."

Edwards said Donna was dedicated and eager to work with and assist the children. She described Donna as "an outstanding person. She is so remarkable in her attitude toward the children and everyone else.

"Donna is a very loving person. She showed everyone else how much she loved them."

Edwards remembered Donna constantly buying the children gifts and always giving to the children. "She was an inspiration to me and to everyone else," she said. "She was an intelligent human being and caught on quite well. As I said before, she seemed to almost read your mind.

"When Donna retired, the entire faculty missed her. I still miss her. She is just a very giving, warm person."

Suzanne Huffman was one of the Coralwood secretaries during Donna's tenure. She said Donna was an amazing person. In fact Huffman went by the nickname, "Office Mama." "I remember when she came in for the first time I didn't think she would be able to do anything. She was wonderful from the start. I could never understand how she could read lips. She was just a dear, dear person. She always kept on plugging. The children flocked to her wherever she was. I remember one time I was sitting at my desk with a disgusted expression and she knew. She always had such a good sense of humor."

When Donna decided to retire from Coralwood, the staff and children were heartbroken, but proud of what she had accomplished for the school. Donna's retirement party in November 1985 was an emotional event, Marcelle recalled, and she received many nice gifts from the parents and children at Coralwood.

Perhaps the highlight of the party was placing the plaque on the library door with Donna's name on it. "We were so proud," Marcelle said.

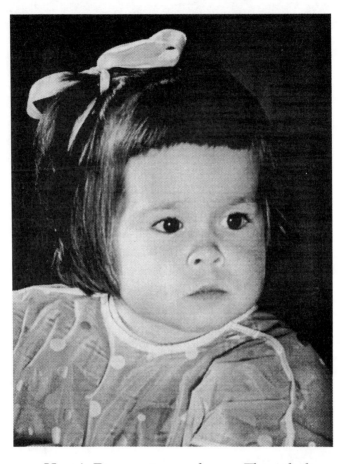

Here is Donna at an early age. Though there may not be any outward signs of her affliction, you can certainly tell she will be an extraordinary child.

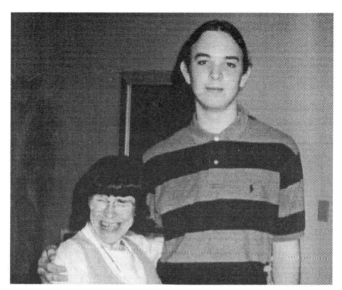

Here's Donna with her nephew Brandon –
who is quite a lad himself.

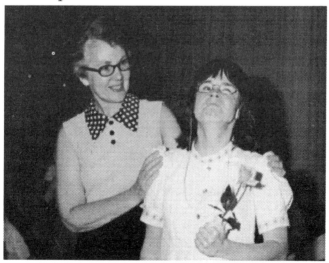

A joyous day in Donna's life – her
graduation from GSD in May 1974.

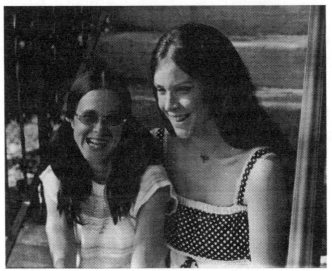

Donna (left) and her sister, Michele, have always shared a very close bond.

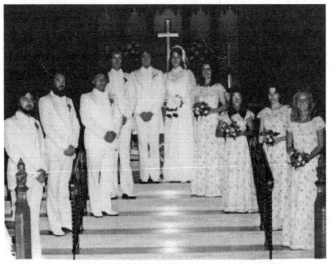

Michele's wedding day – Donna (third from right) served as a bridesmaid.

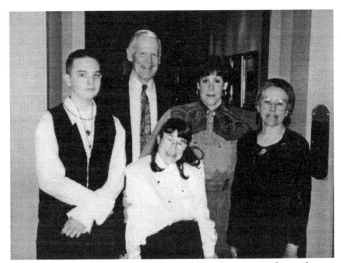

Donna (center) and her loving family – clockwise from left: Brandon, Don, Michele and Marcelle.

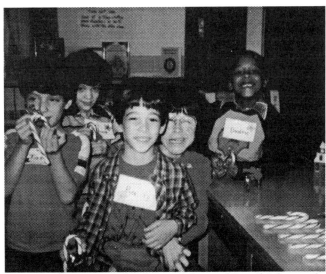

Donna never had trouble making kids smile when she was at the Coralwood Center.

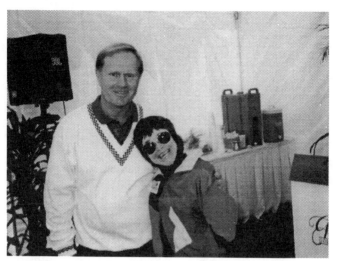

Donna and golfing great Jack Nicklaus first met in South Carolina years ago, and since then, they have struck a good friendship.

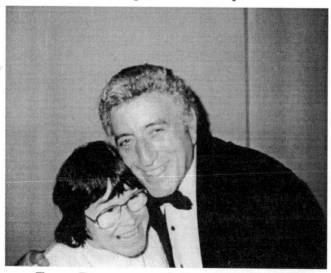

Tony Bennett and Donna, along with Donna's mother, have been friends for years.

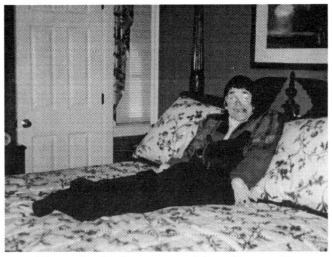

Though she has several handicaps, Donna still manages to live a fairly independent life. Even having her own bed means a lot to her.

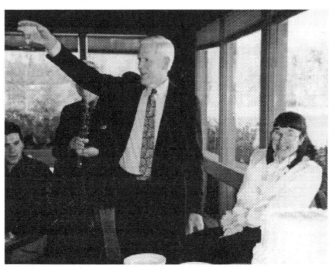

Don (left) gives his daughter a toast at her 40th birthday party. May she have many more!

Chapter 10

Departing is Such
Sweet Sorrow

UTHOR'S NOTE: When
Donna retired in 1985 from
the Coralwood Center, a
school for children with learning
disabilities in DeKalb County, Ga., the joy and
love she brought to the facility made an im-
pression on faculty, staff and students alike.
Here is a sampling of letters and notes written to Donna prior to her departure.)

Dear Donna:

I certainly regretted to learn that it is necessary for you to resign your position at the
Coralwood Center effective Nov. 8, 1985. I have
observed you in the performance of your duties
over the past years and I am appreciative of the
contributions you have made to the Coralwood
Center and the DeKalb County School System.

I wish you good health and happiness in your

future endeavors, and I will always consider you and your parents as good friends of the DeKalb County School System.

Sincerely yours,
York Hudgins
Director
Department of Special Services
DeKalb County School System
Scottdale, Ga.

Dear Donna,

How I will miss you! Your cheerfulness and thoughtfulness are such a big part of life at Coralwood. I am so lucky to have known you and had you as a friend. Come back to see us often.

I know you will always remember your friends at Coralwood as we will remember you. We'll have to have a Coralwood reunion in South Carolina.

Enjoy your leisure and stay well.

Love, Jackie

Dear Donna,

Coralwood won't be Coralwood without you! You've always been there for us when we needed you and when the children needed you. (Don't forget T.J., Teresa or Andy!)

You are a terrific lady who has taught me a great deal. I enjoyed learning to sign with you, even though I am not very good!

Enjoy your leisure time and visit us often!
With love, Cathy

P.S. *Who will fix my chocolate chip cookies now?!?!!??*

Dearest Donna:

After reading all these wonderful notes from all your wonderful friends, I could not elaborate. I have many of the same feelings, but this book is too small for me to itemize the many reasons why you will be missed here at Coralwood.

I remember well the day you and your sweet Mom walked into my office at Doraville. Little did I know that twelve years later, you would still be working with these children. You have done so much to help them and they love you so much.

You have been such a very important member of our staff and a very dear friend to me. I will never understand how you read my lips and my mind at the same time!

Your ability to communicate with others is re-markable. You do a better job than many people without an apparent handicap.

We love you, and will miss you here, but plan to see you often so this is not "goodbye."

Love from your "oldest" friend forever -
Suzanne Huffman

Dear Donna:
In the short time I have been here, I have seen how much you do for everyone - we will really miss you!

Thanks for waiting almost every day for my lunch count. You have been so patient!!

I'll always remember you and the wonderful example you set for us!
Love,
Cathy Schulte

Donna,
You have taught and shown me so much about life - I'll always remember you.

Enjoy your retirement and don't ever stop baking your wonderful chocolate chip cookies!
Love, Phyllis

Dear Donna,
I will miss your smiling face in the halls - but I will always be reminded of you when I sign-in every morning with my "Cindy" magnet.

Good luck and enjoy your leisure time!
Cindy Stein

Donna,
You are really going to be missed! I especially like the way you love the children. I know they

love you back, too!

Thanks for all the last-minute mimeographs (I can never get organized the day before!).

I don't know how bus duty will make it without you. You are such an asset to Coralwood, and there will be more than an empty space when you leave. Once again, you will be missed.

Love,
Helen

Dear Donna -

You are such a special person. Here at Coralwood, you fill such an important need - keeping the teachers "in line" in the library, and giving the children "warm fuzzies."

When you see them in the halls, you see such an important part of the Coralwood family.

We will miss you.

Love,
Betsy

Dear Donna,

I will miss you very much. After all, who will help me to laugh at my mistakes!

I wish you the best in all you do. Keep on being happy and spreading your joy. Enjoy your retirement.

Love ya!

Ava Mason

Oh Donna -

It took me so long to really get to know you and now, I feel awful thinking of "my" hallway without you in it.

I will miss your eyes smiling at me; I will miss the warm smiling at me; I will miss the warm pats on days when I feel "in the dumps" and you seem to be the only one able to inside me; I will miss the reports you give me daily on my children - I'll never be able to send them to the bathroom alone; I will miss using what little sign language I know. But most of all, I'll miss you - the neat, wonderful person I think you are. You've taught me so much and I have grown because I was lucky enough to call you, "Friend."

Much Love, Andee

P.S. *Bless and hug your mom for bringing you into this world and for sharing you with us!*

Chapter 11

"I Left My Heart..."

Long Island, N.Y., has produced many great persons over the years. Marcelle recalls one particular person who has become, as of late, an icon of the MTV generation - singer Tony Bennett, whose most famous song is the standard *I Left My Heart in San Francisco*.

Marcelle, in fact, knew Tony Bennett before he became *the* Tony Bennett. The two grew up in the Long Island town of Astoria nearly 60 years ago and have been friends since childhood.

"He was very devoted to his singing," Marcelle recalled. "He had to give up a lot of opportunities to do things with the kids in the neighborhood because he was always busy with his singing. He had an absolutely beautiful voice; he even sang to my grandmother."

Donna met Marcelle's childhood friend when she was quite young in California; he was performing in a concert at that time. Tony even sang his trademark song at that particular performance, and Marcelle said that he had better put that on a record.

The Gustavels believe Bennett is a very giving and caring person.

A few years ago, Bennett was on a national concert tour and was booked to perform at the Peace Center performing arts facility in Greenville, S.C. Bennett made sure the Gustavels had prime seats for the concert.

During the concert, Bennett dedicated two of his songs to Donna, which she regards to this day as one of her lifetime thrills.

"We were sitting in the side seats because it was easier for Donna to look down on him," Marcelle recalled. "He sang the two songs to her, and when he left the stage, he turned to her and gave her a big wave. It was her big moment. She was very emotional that night, and proud."

After the concert, Bennett wasn't through with his wonderful surprises. He arranged for a white limousine ride for Donna and Marcelle through the city streets of Greenville to a private gathering at the 858 Club in downtown Greenville. The Gustavels had a lengthy visit with Bennett and his drummer Clayton Cameron that evening.

"It was quite a thrill," Donna said. "I will always remember it."

Through the years, Bennett and the Gustavels have corresponded. Bennett never forgets Donna during the holiday season and has sent her many beautiful cards.

Over the years, Tony has sent Donna countless cards and T-shirts. Perhaps the most endearing gift was one of Bennett's art books. Donna and Marcelle said the art book was absolutely gorgeous and they treasured receiving it from the legendary star.

Tony Bennett's signature song has become the theme song for the city of San Francisco, and his many other hits have provided the soundtrack for lovers of all ages.

But to Donna Gustavel and her family, Tony Bennett is one of those loyal friends who has never forgotten his early upbringing.

"Tony has not forgotten his roots," Marcelle said. "He is the same person today as he was when he was a kid. He has changed a little bit, but he is just as kind today as he was then. I have never heard him speak ill about a soul."

Donna was elated when Tony sang to her that night in Greenville. "I can see him singing, and people love him," Donna said. "All the young people love him and love to listen to him."

Dan Brannan

About the limo ride that night, Donna said, "that was the first time I had ridden in a limo; the only other time was when I was a bridesmaid at my sister's wedding."

The Gustavels said they have a lot of respect, adoration and love for the Ralph Sharon Trio, Bennett's musicians, and their music.

Chapter 12

Celebrity Corner

Many of us dream of meeting our favorite celebrities. Unfortunately, most of the time, the only way we get to see them is by watching TV or going to the movies.

Sometimes, we will even write to our favorites, asking for an autograph or a picture. Most of the time, a star's publicist or personal secretary handles the request with an autographed picture or a form letter.

Donna Gustavel has been lucky with celebrities in her life. She has received personal notes from actor Carroll O'Connor (*All in the Family, In the Heat of the Night*), from Charles Schulz (creator of the classic comic strip *Peanuts*) and from a person some believe is the greatest golfer of all time - "The Golden Bear" himself, Jack Nicklaus.

Dan Brannan

Donna's longest-running celebrity relationship, other than with Tony Bennett, has been with
Nicklaus. The Gustavel family first met Nicklaus
in the fall of 1992 at Great Waters Golf Course, a
course he designed, which is located at Reynolds
Plantation in Georgia. They met Nicklaus following a buffet dinner at the club. Nicklaus was impressed that Donna instantly knew him.

"She was just all smiles, and he was just very
nice to her," Marcelle. "Jack Nicklaus is a really kind person and enjoys talking to people."

At their next encounter, Donna gave Nicklaus
some of her chocolate chip cookies. "His family
was with him, and they were all crazy about the
cookies," Marcelle said.

Donna recalled two meetings with Nicklaus
and how she was ready with her cookies when
they met the second time. During that meeting,
she had a picture taken with the legendary golfer.
Today, Donna avidly follows Nicklaus on the Se-
nior PGA Tour and in the Grand Slam events.

Anytime Donna gets a letter from Jack,
she lets out a scream and lets everyone know
it is from him before she opens the letter.
"Jack is a very wonderful and warm person,"
Donna said. "When I first met him, he seemed
very interested in talking with me. He is a
big golf talker."

Here is an example of some of the letters the two have exchanged over the years:

"Thank you for coming out to see me at the opening of Grand Waters last Friday. I enjoyed seeing you and hope you had a good time.

"I also want to thank you for the bag of cookies you gave me. They sure were good!

"I hope our paths cross again some day. Until then, all the best.

**"Sincerely,
Jack Nicklaus."**

"Dear Donna:

"Please excuse me for not dropping you a note sooner. I have rarely been home for more than a day or two at a time this summer, which makes keeping up with my correspondence very difficult. However, I did get your cookies, and they were as great as ever.

"I was delighted to see the nice chapter about you in Dan Brannan's book, Everyday Angels. *Thank you for sending me your autographed copy. It is a welcomed addition to our library.*

"Thanks again for thinking of me, Donna, and please give my regards to your parents.

**"Your friend,
Jack Nicklaus."**

Dan Brannan

Donna's friendship with Schulz began when Harry Layne, a Keowee Key, S.C., resident who is a close friend of Schulz, told him of Donna's love for *Peanuts* and Snoopy while he was on a trip to California. "Donna sent to Schulz the pictures of what she did with Snoopy while with the children at Coralwood," Marcelle said. "She had Snoopy placemats at the school and had always loved Snoopy. When she was a child, anytime she had to do something on the wall, she did Snoopy; she absolutely loved him."

Schulz wrote back and sent Donna a drawing of his cartoon beagle sleeping on top of his doghouse, along with a card. "She was just thrilled," Marcelle said.

Schulz's letter went like this:

"Thank you for the wonderful drawings of Snoopy. The enclosed photograph of you reflects such a happy smile which is no doubt why you gave Snoopy such a happy expression, too.

"I'm very pleased to know that Snoopy brings you such enjoyment, and I appreciate your taking the time to prepare and send me your drawings.

"Kindest regards,
Charles M. Schulz."

Donna came in contact with O'Connor for the first time while O'Connor was hospitalized at Emory University Hospital in Atlanta. He was filming the television series *In The Heat of the Night* at the time in Georgia and was on the same floor as Don when he had to have heart surgery.

Donna met him while on one of her visits to Don and later sent him a get-well card. O'Connor responded in the following way:

"I'd like to write something special, like the fond message you wrote to me, but by the time my special replies reached all the thousands of sweet well-wishers, hardly anyone would remember what the crisis was about. Better to say as soon as possible the same words of thanks to everybody.

"God bless you for your loving thoughts and prayers; they made the good things happen for me and Nancy and Hugh.

"Love from Carroll."

Chapter 13

One Big, Happy Family

In situations like the one the Gustavel family endures, there are times that jealousy and other problems can arise among siblings.

Although that was the case at times, the Gustavel daughters, Donna and Michele, sincerely love and care for each other. Michele loves Donna so much that when she was married, she chose Donna as a bridesmaid. Donna proudly walked down the aisle all by herself.

Michele was a year-and-a-half old when Donna was born. Marcelle and Don always felt it was important to do as much for Michele as for Donna. Marcelle said Don was very helpful in making sure things were balanced and good for both girls.

Michele today is 44 and lives in St. Simons Island, Ga. She believes that her family has always been a normal type of family. Michele says she and Donna are very close.

"She is so intuitive," Michele said, "and anticipates what to do and say. We had our times when we didn't get along, like any other siblings, but we both had very happy childhoods and were happy children.

"We got a lot of our parents' strength and faith. They are extremely strong individuals."

Michele is an interior decorator and lives with her 17-year-old son, Brandon.

"Donna and Brandon are extremely close and have had a solid bond from the beginning," Michele said. "That is the way it has always been. They almost don't have to speak.

"We did finger-spell and sign language at an early age. It's like getting up and brushing our teeth."

Michele is very proud of Donna's ability as an aunt. She said Donna has been outstanding with Brandon. "Donna has been a whole lot of fun," Michele said.

Michele believes Donna is extremely intelligent. "It's hard for me to hear her referred to as 'retarded,'" Michele said. "She is so smart. It really irritates me for people to think she doesn't have a brain.

"Because of Donna's deafness, I think I look more at what is inside of people. She is so in tune with everything. She doesn't have psychic ability, but she has something beyond normal intuitive abilities."

At times, Donna's condition has made Michele sad. "It's a shame she is so physically afflicted," Michele said. "With a simple blood exchange, her life could have been so much different."

Michele believes she is more like her father, a very serious person. "I've been through several things in my life, such as cancer, and always had Donna's support in my ups and downs," Michele said. "She always keeps me smiling. She is very sensitive to other people's needs. Her feelings can be hurt. You have to be very careful not to ever talk about her in a negative way because she is very perceptive and can read lips.

"She can tell immediately if I'm up or down. We've always helped motivate each other. When I am down, Donna helps me get up and vice versa."

Michele is sometimes jealous of the time Donna gets to spend with her parents. "I wish I could spend more time with my parents," Michele said. "My mother is a very deep, sensitive, caring person. She is very emotional and a very intelligent person. She is an absolute ball to be around."

When Michele developed a tumor in her salivary glands in 1975, she had to undergo deep radiology treatment. Her family and Donna were always there, encouraging her.

Michele is also very physically fit, running and working out like her sister. One of Michele's friends, John O'Connell, is a certified athletic trainer at Southeast Georgia Regional Hospital. He, too, is amazed at Donna's ability to use her body in workouts after all the physical problems she has. Michele believes that the workouts have helped better Donna's quality of life.

"She was always told she would never do this or that," Michele said. "But her body is like an athletic body."

Donna said she loves Michele and worries about her. "I try to do whatever I can to help her," she said. "I care very much about Michele."

Thanks to the Gustavels' efforts, Michele and Donna have a beautiful relationship. Each sister is always there for the other, and Donna always brightens her sister's life.

Chapter 14

Someone to Lean On

Most families might find that having a son or daughter who is handicapped a hindrance to strong intra-family relationships.

Of course, the Gustavel family is not the typical family.

The bond between Donna and her nephew, Brandon Morgan, began when Brandon was but an infant, the newborn son of her sister, Michele. Donna remembered Brandon as being a lot of fun when he was small.

"I used to feed him," she said. "I'd play with him, and when he was naughty, I would scold him."

Today, Donna perceives Brandon as tall and grown up. "He works very hard, and I'm proud of that," Donna said. "He is a cook at a restaurant."

One of Brandon's proudest moments occurred recently when he served Donna and the entire Gustavel family at Allegro's in St. Simons Island. "They were on their way to a vacation cruise when they stopped and ate at the restaurant," Brandon remarked. "When I served them, Donna was almost in tears. She was so proud of me."

Donna said Brandon is a sweet boy, although she is not hesitant to tell him when she doesn't like something he does.

Donna has always been supportive of Brandon, making sure he got excellent Christmas and birthday gifts. One year, Donna got him a Nintendo video game system. She also has given him various Snoopy items.

"Donna has always been there for Brandon," Marcelle said. "She's given him nice things and has had a lot of fun with him. Brandon is very protective of Donna."

Brandon feels Donna has been a special person. He says he has always gotten along with his aunt. "I'm her only nephew," he said, "I don't know a lot of sign language, but we still communicate very well. She picks up on what I'm saying well. She has been doing that all my life.

"She reads people's lips well. If people are talking about her, she probably can read their lips."

Brandon sees Donna as being a very loving and caring person. She never forgets anything. "If I send her a card, she will never forget it," Brandon said.

Brandon himself has a seizure disorder and feels his aunt's battle with cerebral palsy and deafness has inspired him. "She has to take things day-by-day," Brandon said. "It's not easy for her."

Brandon says his relationship with his aunt has grown through the years. "I have grown up and am a lot more mature now," he said. "I'm not such a brat anymore. I have never had any problem communicating with Donna, even though Donna can't speak. I don't know what made it so easy. I feel like she can almost read minds. She is very intelligent.

"I definitely think she knows what is going on at all times. If something has gone bad, she immediately knows it."

One of the most special things about Donna and Brandon's relationship is that Donna has always been someone Brandon can lean on in difficult times. "We lived in Seneca (S.C.) when I was about 10, and we went over to her house all the time," Brandon said. "We read things, watched TV and had a lot of fun.

"She is very special."

Chapter 15

Exercising the Right

When Bill Clinton was re-elected as president of the United States in November 1996, one person in a voting booth that day was 41-year-old Donna Gustavel.

Donna is a firm believer in exercising the franchise. She began voting in her early 20s and has always believed it was important.

Marcelle says, "Donna has never missed an election."

Don has always been wise about politics with his many successful years in the business world. He says the Gustavel family has always had a number of discussions about politics, and he feels he and Marcelle have influenced Donna in her urge to vote.

Don and Marcelle do not attempt to tell Donna who to support politically. They prefer that she makes up her own mind. "She forms her own opinions from what she sees on TV and what she sees in newspapers," Don said. "She also observes public reaction to politicians and political situations."

Marcelle says that Don has worked diligently to make sure Donna has all her questions answered about politicians. "She never misses voting," Marcelle said. "She is very smart about the election process. We always vote in the Stamp Creek precinct, which represents Keowee Key. They have a lot of the same volunteers who work each election year in and year out. All the volunteers know Donna."

Donna says she studies the personalities of the candidates and wants to choose a person based on his or her character and what he or she represents.

The Gustavels used to have a closed-captioned television, but found it too difficult for Donna to keep up with the material. Today, she watches the politicians on TV and reads their lips for their statements.

Donna's favorite politician is the same as that of many others in the Oconee County, S.C., area - South Carolina State Sen. Thomas Alexander, who represents Oconee County and Clemson in the state Senate in Columbia.

She has met Alexander on several occasions and believes he is a good person. Alexander is one of the area's most popular politicians and works to help improve the quality of life for all people, regardless of political persuasion.

Donna has always been keenly interested in the presidential and vice-presidential candidates, but does not follow the typical party-line philosophy of voting. Instead, she makes her selections, based on the person, not ideology. She basically votes for who she believes would be a good leader.

Unlike many who believe voting is a waste of time, Donna takes her right to vote seriously. She wishes more people would come out to the polls each election day instead of staying home.

Chapter 16

It's Not Always Fun

W hen Donna was a small child, she came to the realization that she was different than other children. Marcelle remembered that day vividly.

"Donna had been crossing the street, and some other girls looked over and nearly stared holes through her," Marcelle said.

Marcelle remembered telling Donna that they were looking at her beautiful, long and flowing hair.

When Donna was 5 or 6, one day, out of the blue, she confronted Marcelle again. This time, she wanted to know what was really different about herself.

Marcelle told her, then explained how she had cerebral palsy since birth and how she needed a blood exchange to survive, but it had not been done in time. Donna was pleased to know the truth.

Many children are afraid of Donna when they first see her and have to warm up to her. "She smiles at them, and sometimes, she gets a smile back," Marcelle said. "She doesn't push herself on children. She gives them time to warm up. She really loves children."

Inside, Marcelle says she knows Donna hurts whenever people stare at her, whether it is in a store or on the street. Marcelle remembered one incident when two brothers passed Donna in a grocery store. One of the brothers was considerably older than the other.

The younger boy began to laugh and cut up about Donna. "I think I saw stars that day," Marcelle said. "I said to the boy, 'That's not funny, and you shouldn't look at people that way.'

"The older boy was embarrassed at how his brother had acted. The mother didn't do anything about the child's behavior, either, which also bothered me. Donna just kept on moving along with her head held up high that day."

Another time, Donna and Marcelle met a family that kept stopping and staring at her at each aisle. "Sometimes, if it hits me wrong, I'll lose my temper," Marcelle said. "Michele really gets mad about it if someone is staring at Donna. She will sometimes blow her top. Donna just ignores it. She doesn't want to make a scene.

"Some people just aren't tuned in and show a lack of education. We get this a lot in grocery stores, especially on weekends, or if we go to a city like Greenville (S.C.) and go to the mall. Donna feels more secure when she is walking with her father when she is in the mall."

People often say things that are inappropriate about handicapped people. Once, Marcelle heard a doctor saying, "You know how these people are," referring to handicapped people in a negative way. Marcelle said she was steamed about that incident. Donna, though, always tries to keep her head high and not let people's bad intentions get to her.

"I don't want any tears or crying for me because of my handicaps," Donna said. "Push your sadness away if you have any sadness about me. I am happy. If someone stares at me, I will often try to hug them or smile at them."

That smile often melts the barrier between Donna and the starer.

Perhaps that is the best way to break down barriers between those who are handicapped and those who are not - one person at a time.

Chapter 17

Those World- Famous Cookies

One of Donna's favorite pastimes is baking. One of her favorite foods to bake is chocolate chip cookies. These cookies have become well-known, not only to Donna's friends at Keowee Key, but also have become famous across the country thanks to the many celebrities for whom she has baked, celebrities such as Tony Bennett and Jack Nicklaus.

Almost anyone can bake chocolate chip cookies, but Donna adds a special magical touch to them that makes them stand out from all the rest. The reason these cookies are so tasty is because they are made from scratch with Donna's own recipe.

She measures out all the ingredients and handles everything involved in the baking process, except for the actual placement of the cookies into the hot oven. Marcelle or Don handles that task.

The cookies are expensive to make, but are worth every penny she invests. A batch of cookies is packed with raisins, chocolate chips and nuts. Donna actually mixes the ingredients and refuses to use anything less than top-quality ingredients.

The Gustavel's freezer, for years, has been packed with pre-made chocolate chip cookies. Donna spoils father Don by keeping him a separate stash of the legendary delights. "Father's cookies always come first," Marcelle said. "Nobody touches his cookies!"

Donna is an excellent cook and loves spending time in the kitchen."Donna makes excellent pumpkin bread and banana nut bread," Marcelle said.

If Marcelle makes a mistake when cooking, Donna immediately notices. "When Donna was at Coralwood, she spoiled the children constantly with her cookies," Marcelle said.

Nicklaus is one of Donna's biggest chocolate chip cookie fans. In fact, when Nicklaus talks about her cookies, Donna erupts with excitement.

A few of Donna's friends in Atlanta have her recipe. Although they have tried, none of them have succeeded in working the magic Donna has with these delights. Marcelle may have an explanation for it:

"It is probably because Donna compensates some because of her lack of hearing and can concentrate fully on what she is doing," she said. "When we are making the cookies, the phone rings or we are always busy doing other things. But when she makes her cookies, they require her full attention."

Chapter 18

Life at Keowee Key

At its surface, Keowee Key is a collection of lovely homes surrounded by a body of water, Lake Keowee. The scenery is beautiful, and the area is considered one of the most pristine environments in the United States.

But at its heart, Keowee Key is really people, people who have decided to spend their retirement years at this venue.

Donna and her family arrived here in 1985. The Gustavels began commuting to Keowee Key in 1983 before moving two years later. The entire family fell in love with the lake, the area and the people.

"It's very pretty here," Donna said. "I don't do all the things I used to before we moved here. I used to get around more, and I met a lot of people. I have had to slow down some because of the cerebral palsy.

"I am very happy here. I am so comfortable with the stores."

"We have loved it at Keowee Key," Marcelle said. "We have a good time here. Donna knows a lot of people and feels comfortable here. She loves her neighbors and is invited to a lot of parties.

"We love the lake, although we have never had a boat. We have been on a lot of other people's boats, though."

The list of people Donna has come into contact with at Keowee Key is endless, and all of her friends could never be mentioned in one place. Suffice it to say, however, that Donna has touched many lives since moving to the area so many years ago.

When Donna isn't making a trip to the Kourthouse Fitness Center, she is gardening, cooking, visiting neighbors, attending parties or walking near Lake Keowee.

One of Donna's favorite pastimes now is collecting empty cans, which comes partially out of her love for, and efforts to protect, the environment through recycling.

Don takes Donna to nearby Clemson, S.C., to recycle the cans. "Many people drop off cans at the house when they have them," Marcelle said.

"We collect them and take them to Clemson."

Donna has a can party each year. She invites the people who give her cans and has a little party for them, a luncheon, cocktail party or dinner. She plans it and does it all.

One of the reasons Donna probably started accumulating cans is her love for Tab, Coca-Cola's pioneering diet cola. Today, the product is difficult to find throughout the nation. Most Tab sales are concentrated in Coke's home Southeastern territory.

Don has often driven as far as Coke's hometown of Atlanta to cart several cases of the drink back home. Today, Don gets it wherever he can find it, usually in drugstores in Greenville and Anderson, S.C.

Another Keowee Key resident, Harry Layne, was responsible for introducing Donna to one of her celebrity friends - *Peanuts* creator Charles Schulz. Layne first met Donna about 10 years ago through social settings.

"Anyone who knows her loves her," Layne said. "She loves to take care of her dog, Luv."

"Don and Marcelle have given their lives for Donna. Donna loves cruises and getting on a ship. Because of Don and Marcelle's support, they have made a good life for her and for each other."

Next-door neighbors Lorraine and Bill

Barber have known Donna for four years. Lorraine describes Donna as "one of the most thoughtful and sweetest people I have ever met." "I have a granddaughter who came here last fall. While she was here, Donna got her a white teddy bear.

"She always has to invite us over. I know she has a lot of pain, but she never talks about it. Her parents are very devoted. They are great with her.

"When they are visiting, and Donna is ready to go home, they take her back. Donna reads lips well. She laughs at some things, and you can tell she is astute. She is a smart girl. She loves to cook and always has cake and cookies available."

Lorraine was a nurse at one time, so she makes sure she doesn't squeeze Donna too tight because of her muscular difficulties.

"Donna is one of the few people with cerebral palsy who hasn't gone into a wheelchair," Lorraine said. "She is determined not to let that happen. Many cerebral palsy children are in a wheelchair by age 6 or 7. Donna didn't let that happen to her."

J.R. Riggs and his wife, Dorothy, have been two of Donna's longest neighbors. He says he has known the Gustavels for about 15 years. "That young lady is thoughtful of other people, more than she is about herself," Riggs said. "She loves people and loves to be around them. She is considerate and loves my grandchildren. I don't know a neighbor or person out here who doesn't think she's an angel.

"We had a German shepherd once that she thought the world of. She was as upset as we were when it died. We enjoy having her as a friend and neighbor. Once you meet her, I don't know of anyone who won't go out of his or her way to do things for her. Our grandchildren love her and always ask about her. She really has an impact on people. If you are not feeling well, she makes you feel better."

When *Everyday Angels* was released, the Riggs' daughter, Cathee Stegall, called to say she read about Donna in her church's copy of the book. J.R. went out and bought a book for himself. "This is just what people think about Donna. She is a great inspiration to everyone, from small children to adults," Riggs said. "The first time they came here, they were still living in Atlanta. We were the only two houses in our district at the time. I went in, and her mother and father asked me if I wanted something to drink.

"From then on, that drink is what I got when Donna was there. She never forgets anything. Donna has a love for animals, too, especially her little Chihuahua, Luv. When we had the German shepherd, my wife got a statue of a German shepherd and we gave it to her.

"Two years ago, when she got her dog, my wife saw a little 2-3 inch perfect statue of a Chihuahua. We gave it to her. The German shepherd is now on her dresser with a photograph of her family and the Chihuahua statue. That is how positive she thinks of other people."

Dick and Marie Warner are other neighbors who have known Donna for about eight years. Marie views Donna as a special individual who adds a lot of smiles to other people's lives.

"It is unbelievable the things she does, and she makes you aware of how special she is," Marie said. "My heart just melts when I see her. I can't completely explain it. She and her parents are very special people. They make you aware of what life is all about. She always has a smile on her face. Donna is so outgoing.

"Donna, Marcelle and I had surgery about the same time several years ago. The operations seemed to bond us all. We feel blessed that we have gotten to know her."

Marie's husband, Dick, says Donna is one of the most special people he has ever met. "I never saw anyone as upbeat and positive as she," Dick said. "She has two exceptional parents. They have a very close-knit family. I am very proud to have them as friends.

"They have a lot of love for her, and she shows a lot of love back to them."

Dr. Ronald Moore has been Donna's dentist since she came to Keowee Key. He says Donna has a certain spark about her. "She is so positive," he said. "The three of them always brighten things up for me and my staff when they come in. I think a lot of her."

Gayle Lusk first met Donna when she worked at the Kourthouse Fitness Center. Donna and Gayle first communicated on paper, and eventually, Gayle learned some sign language so they could communicate easier. Gayle says that Donna has helped put her life in perspective.

"We tend to take a lot for granted," Gayle said. "By watching Donna, you can see better what is involved in life. We take our health, communicating and a lot of things for granted. I don't think she realizes what a difference she has made in my life. She is really special.

"Even though she may not be able to communicate verbally, she is still able to communicate. We have inside jokes and laugh about things. I would think she inspires anyone who has ever met her. I don't think there is anything she can't do."

Gayle remembers many people coming into

the Kourthouse and complaining of small aches and pains. However, Donna keeps going with her head up high and smiling, even if she isn't feeling well.

"She's the most incredible person that I know," Gayle said.

Donna remembers going shopping in Greenville, S.C., one time near her parents' anniversary. She put together an incredible bouquet of flowers, picking out each individual flower.

"Donna has a fantastic sense of humor," Lusk said, "and it is always fun being with her. Donna has had a spectacular life. She is much loved by everybody who has ever come into contact with her at Lake Keowee."

Donna's popularity at Keowee Key is universal. In fact, during the Christmas season of 1996, one of Donna's neighbors marked the 12-day period to the holiday with a series of messages, the first of which read like this:

"Twas the first night of Christmas, and all thru your house
Not a creature was stirring, not even a mouse.
Except suddenly, one little soul did appear
It's your 'CHRISTMAS FRIEND' who brings

holiday cheer.

"Tonite it's a partridge for your pear tree
And tomorrow, who knows, you must wait
and see.
So hang out your stocking each nite with care
(as soon after 5 p.m. as possible)
And you know your 'CHRISTMAS FRIEND'
soon will be there.

"Be aware of this warning: Your friend will
be here
But don't try to catch him, or he'll disappear."
Your Christmas Friend.

Each day, Donna left a stocking outside the house. The neighbor would then come by and leave a surprise. Donna tried to figure out who the person was, but remained surprised throughout the adventure. She was grateful, though, for the gesture.

Chapter 19

On the Road Again

Marcelle and Don Gustavel have always enjoyed traveling, but have refused to do it without Donna at their sides. Many people with cerebral palsy or multiple handicaps don't get to experience the things Donna has been able to over the years. Donna has visited the Caribbean, Europe and Mexico and has traveled throughout most of the United States, including Alaska and Hawaii.

Donna has loved each and every trip. Many of these trips have been cruises. During each cruise, the captains have fallen in love with Donna and allowed her to visit the bridge of each ship. She has seen sights from a captain's view that many people never get to experience.

"Donna especially enjoyed Captain Young on the Alaska trip," Marcelle said. "She really got to know him. She loved Alaska and also flying on board (the supersonic jetliner) Concorde in Europe.

"She loved Hawaii, but we had some bad weather while we were there."

The last trip the Gustavels made was a jazz cruise in the Caribbean. "The couple with whom we traveled, Jane and John MacAuley, were fantastic," Marcelle said. "They kept Donna laughing and having a wonderful time throughout the trip. The captain was very good to her and everyone else was so nice to her."

As Donna slows down physically, it has become harder for the Gustavels to travel.

"When Donna and Michele were younger, they made many trips up and down California, so Donna basically has always traveled," said Marcelle.

"Donna really loves to go to different places. She has sometimes had trouble riding in a car and could barely lie down because of her back problems, but she usually does very well on long trips to places like Florida. I think the exercise helps her as far as traveling goes because it keeps her more flexible."

Don counted that the family has been on 12 total cruises. "We have always had a ball with Donna," he said. "We have included her on all our trips. The trips to Hawaii and Tahiti were difficult, but we toughed it out."

The Gustavels are uncertain how much more they will travel in the future as they get older, but they will always have the memories of the many cruises, and Donna will always remember seeing places and experiencing things people with multiple handicaps do not ordinarily get to do.

Don and Marcelle certainly are examples for parents of handicapped children to follow. Rather than excluding their child because of the possible problems they may encounter, Don and Marcelle have enthusiastically included Donna in all their plans.

If only other parents would do the same for their children.

Chapter 20

The Big 4-0

A 40th birthday is always a significant milestone in any person's life. When Donna turned 40 on Feb. 16, 1994, the celebration became doubly important.

Reason: Most people with cerebral palsy don't live much past 20 years. Donna had beaten all the odds by reaching 40.

Donna had made her mind up long before turning 40 that she was going to have a big birthday bash. In her normal, independent style, Donna paid for the entire gathering at the Keowee Key Conference Center.

She also planned the entire event, selecting her guest list, picking out the menu and even deciding what kind of cake would be served.

A little more than 100 people were invited and most of them came. Jack Nicklaus and Tony Bennett could not attend, owing to previous commitments, but both sent best wishes to Donna.

People came from all over for her party. A former schoolteacher came as did several friends from the Atlanta area. The birthday party was one of Don and Marcelle's proudest moments for Donna.

"She does all the details for her parties," Don said. "This was a very proud night for all of us."

Marcelle added, "The 40th birthday party was a good time to reflect on everything Donna had done in her lifetime. I thought about all the years and all the things we had done and gone through. We always took it one day at a time.

"When she turned 40, I looked back and wondered how we did it. There was a lot of work involved for all of us. There were so many people who contributed and shared and helped make her what she is today."

Bennett placed a personal phone call to Donna, letting her know he couldn't come that night. "The call was a big thrill," Marcelle said.

Donna said the party was a big thrill and she loved the evening.

Don vividly recalled his toast in front of the large crowd. "Here's to Donna on her 40th!," he said, "and to all of you, and your kindness to her." When Don made the toast that night and said those words, there was hardly a dry eye in the house.

The people in attendance were proud of Donna and the Gustavel family for enabling Donna to make it to her 40th birthday - a milestone, especially for anyone with cerebral palsy.

Chapter 21

Luv Conquers All

Since Donna moved to Keowee Key in 1985, she had always wanted her own dog. She talked and talked with Don persistently, and finally, Don's heart melted. He got her a small Chihuahua.

Donna fell in love with the dog from the very beginning, but wasn't sure what to name it. She did know she wanted to name it something she could pronounce.

The Gustavels proceeded to work on words Donna could say out loud. One of those words was Donna's favorite word, love, which, spelled phonetically, comes out luv.

The name for the dog stuck, and today, Luv is Donna's constant companion, traveling wth her just about everywhere.

Luv will be 3 years old in March 1997 and has brought the Gustavels much happiness. "I love

Luv," Donna said. "I play with her, chase her and throw things to her. She runs around the room fast. I feed Luv pretty good stuff. Luv is paper-trained and is very good about it.

"Luv sleeps in my bedroom, and the door stays open so there are no accidents on my rug."

Donna has long seemed to have a way with animals. Don perceives the communication between Donna and animals as a natural process.

"There is an awareness from Luv of Donna's limitations," Don says, "yet Luv is compelled by Donna's love."

Marcelle agrees that there is a special bond between Donna's dog and her. Luv even seems to know Donna's sign-language.

Luv can constantly be found at Donna's feet. The dog will obey Donna's sign to sit or get down. If Donna is ever gone, Luv immediately runs to her when she returns. It is safe to say that Luv is one of the most spoiled Chihuahuas in all of Keowee Key.

Marcelle carries Luv down the stairs at night rather than having Luv run down the steps.

The relationship between the two is a very special one. If dogs are, in fact, "man's best friend," then Donna certainly has a very special friend in Luv.

Chapter 22

Soldiering On

In the previous chapter, we introduced you to Donna's pet dog, Luv. In many ways, Luv is a pretty appropriate name for this pooch, because love is how the Gustavel family has managed to survive the many crises it has faced over the years.

Don and Marcelle have always felt Donna gives more than she takes from them and consider her a joy to be around. The Gustavels have always had to take things a day and a step at a time.

Long ago, Marcelle said that she and Don put Donna's future in God's hands and that God has never let them down. Marcelle believes that she has constantly been led by a higher power through the many crisis situations they have faced over the years.

"There has definitely been a lot of love in our house," Michele said. "Mom represents everything a mother should be. We always thought we had a normal household. When I left home, it changed things, and our immediate family is very close. We don't have to work hard at it. Everything between us all just comes naturally."

Marcelle says that there are times when she wonders how she and Don have managed to make it through the things they have faced in 40-plus years. "I have no regrets about anything," Marcelle said. "I wouldn't do it any differently. We can't tell other people what to do in the same kind of situations we have faced with Donna's deafness and palsy.

"If people can't cope, then they have to take other steps. The key is to take things a day at a time and not dwell on negative things."

Marcelle believes parents in a similar situation cannot feel sorry for themselves and seek pity from others. "From the moment Donna was born, I loved her and knew she was my responsibility," Marcelle said. "Don has been a wonderful father, and Michele and Brandon have also been wonderful. Don is a very strong man and very understanding."

Again, Marcelle and Don believe that people who cannot handle their children should explore other options. "It has to be up to the individual families," Marcelle said. "Every situation is different. I have no dispute with parents if they decide to do something different than we did. They have to decide what is right for them and their particular situation."

Many parents probably could not handle such a tough assignment as the one Don and Marcelle were given when Donna was born. It certainly takes special people to do what they have done over the years for their daughter, and I have nothing but admiration for the job they have done in raising Donna.

Chapter 23

In Her Own Words

AUTHOR'S NOTE: The following chapter is Donna's story in her own words. As you might be able to tell, she has a unique perspective on her life.

I have had a good life - living as normal a life as possible with cerebral palsy, deafness and no speech. This is my life.

A long time ago, when I was born, I was very sick. The doctors didn't think I would live. Little did they know I was born a fighter.

I survived the very long operation when they did a complete exchange of blood. Shortly after going home, I was diagnosed with CP. Shortly after that, my parents realized I was also deaf.

At the age of 1, I attended a nursery school for children with multiple handicaps. Although the psychologist said my mentality would not go beyond three years, the doctors and staff felt differently. I was eager to learn and to work hard.

My first teacher was amazed at how quickly I learned. My schooling, in the early days, was not that of a deaf child; somehow, my teacher taught me to read and write, to spell and do math.

After school, I would go home and do my homework and study with the help of my mother. The hard work paid off - my grades were A's all through school.

Along with the educational work, there was much physical and occupational therapy. I had to be "trained" to use the muscles in my body to do things many take for granted. Soon, I was able to sit alone, to walk, to dress, to feed myself, plus all the things people can do for themselves, but take for granted. It was again hard work and complete hard work from the staff that helped me.

The school I attended in California was the El Portal Cerebral Palsy School for Handicapped Children. During my last year there, and since then, there have been several children who have been deaf or hard of hearing. A teacher for the deaf was added to the staff. He, too, was deaf - and an excellent teacher.

He loved working with me; he was amazed at how quickly I learned and how eager I was. He felt I was quite bright. This was the feeling of all the staff.

It wasn't all work - there was much fun, too. At school, I was in the plays, I was a cheerleader, I won the dominos championship, played basket-ball and sang with the choir.

I am happy here in Keowee Key. I will live here for the rest of my life. I love my house and people are warm to me. I love everyone. I give hugs; please, don't be sad. If you are sad, you will be better later. Don't be sad, be happy. I will help you if you are sad.

I know the people at the store, and they are nice to me. I have fun at the stores.

It is very pretty here. I go to the Kourthouse all the time. Everyone is nice. I love it. It is safe here; I have lots of friends. People do nice things for me. For example, when I was going on a trip to Hawaii, Bess and Fred Robinson had a big din-ner party for me.

I get invited to parties most of the time. Some-times, I just stay home. Other people do so much for me. I get a lot of thank-you notes and Christ-mas cards.

I hope to stay strong and healthy, and I hope to stay here. I can get help when I need it. I have kept many of my friends. I have an aluminum can party once a year, and I do not have to work

116

anymore; I am retired.

I do try to work in the garden a little, and I continue to go to the spa and exercise. I can't do it like I used to; I know my CP is why. I like trips, and I hope to go on lots more. Later, much later, I would like to see Jack Nicklaus, Tony Bennett and Charles Schulz and hug Carroll O'Connor and tell him not to worry. Someday, I would like to be on Oprah Winfrey's Book Club.

I thank everyone in my life. I will continue to cook and bake a lot and take care of Luv.

Thank you, thank you, Dan Brannan, for caring about me.

Chapter 24

Keeping the Faith

Donna plans a party for her 45th birthday on Feb. 16, 1999. Marcelle is betting she will celebrate her 45th in style and have many more birthdays after that.

"She exercises and is careful about what she eats," Marcelle said.

Still, in the back of her and her family's mind must be the lingering thought of what they would do if something happened to Donna or to them.

Don and Marcelle are both in their early 70s; Don is very concerned with making plans for Donna if something should happen to either him or Marcelle.

"Our concern for Donna is that she would be able to be on her own once we are gone," Don said. "We will not burden Michele. We must find a place where Donna would be happy and self-sufficient. She is very capable of handling her own finances, but has physical problems which prohibit her from being alone.

"We need to get on the ball and make arrangements for her."

With the thought of death also comes the thought of an afterlife.

The Gustavels aren't found in church each week, but definitely believe in God. Donna has a hard time sitting in church pews because of her physical problems. "We went to church until Donna couldn't bear sitting in the church pew anymore," Marcelle said. "Donna has a definite faith in Jesus and loves him.

"Donna is very emotional about Jesus and is very religious. We believe in God very much, and we all pray. Donna has VCR tapes that go through the whole process of the birth of Christ. She gets very emotional about it and tears up when she talks about Christ's birth.

"I think there is a strong relationship between Donna and Jesus. Donna also has a children's Bible she refers to constantly."

Marcelle remembered a time that Donna was having some horrible tests prior to one of her surgeries in the hospital. Once, late at night, Marcelle said she felt a hand on her shoulder, telling her not to worry, that she would get through everything.

"The same thing has happened with Don," Marcelle said. "God has been there when we needed him. We believe very, very strongly in God. I believe God put Donna here to give of her heart and soul to others and to help other people."

When Donna hugs someone, she means it from the bottom of her heart, Marcelle says. "When Donna hugs, she gives," Marcelle added. "She feels she is giving her strength to you. I also feel that she is somehow capable of seeing things before you know it. I believe these are all gifts from God.

"God has given us a lot."

Chapter 25

Conclusion

Growing up as a child in southwestern Illinois, I learned a lot from my own mother and father. One of the key things I learned in the Brannan household was that a person should not judge a book by its cover and always look beneath the exterior before making a final decision about the merit of another person.

I can't think of anyone who better epitomizes the old phrase "never judge a book by its cover" than Donna Gustavel.

Donna Gustavel may look different than you and me; she may be deaf; and she may have a unique gait. But inside, she has an endless amount of energy, enthusiasm, intellect and a zest for life few people can match.

Donna's neighbor, J.R. Riggs, said in his business life, he has known all types of people. He knows one thing for certain: if the world could be made up of people like Donna Gustavel, it certainly would be a different place.

"Donna loves everyone, and everyone loves

her back," Riggs told me when I interviewed him.

I hope that parents of physically challenged children will be inspired after they read *The Courage To Live*. Just because a child is handicapped does not mean they do not have the potential to learn, to expand their horizons and eventually help others who face the same predicament.

The Gustavels are a prime example that parents *can* make the best of life, even if their child is physically and mentally challenged. A child with cerebral palsy does *not* have to be in a wheelchair by the age of 6 or 7.

I think Keowee Key's Harry Layne may have said it best: "When some are complaining of small aches and pains, think about what Donna Gustavel has to face each day."

I hope this book will give you the courage to face the trials in your own life with as much humor and sensitivity as Donna.

Donna Gustavel and her family have shown all of us that she has the compassion, sense of humor and love a person needs to live. But above all, she has the courage to live.